The Plant Based Diet For Beginners

A Complete Diet Guide for Beginners for Easy Weight Loss and Burn Fat to Kick-Start a Healthy Lifestyle

Vegetarian Academy

© Copyright 2020 by Vegetarian Academy - All rights reserved.

The following Book is reproduced below with the goal of providing information that is as accurate and reliable as possible. Regardless, purchasing this Book can be seen as consent to the fact that both the publisher and the author of this book are in no way experts on the topics discussed within and that any recommendations or suggestions that are made herein are for entertainment purposes only. Professionals should be consulted as needed prior to undertaking any of the action endorsed herein.

This declaration is deemed fair and valid by both the American Bar Association and the Committee of Publishers Association and is legally binding throughout the United States.

Furthermore, the transmission, duplication, or reproduction of any of the following work including specific information will be considered an illegal act irrespective of if it is done electronically or in print. This extends to creating a secondary or tertiary copy of the work or a recorded copy and is only allowed with the express written consent from the Publisher. All additional right reserved.

The information in the following pages is broadly considered a truthful and accurate account of facts and as such, any inattention, use, or misuse of the information in question by the reader will render any resulting actions solely under their purview. There are no scenarios in which the publisher or the original author of this work can be in any fashion deemed liable for any hardship or damages that may befall them after undertaking information described herein.

Additionally, the information in the following pages is intended only for informational purposes and should thus be thought of as universal. As befitting its nature, it is presented without assurance regarding its prolonged validity or interim quality. Trademarks that are mentioned are done without written consent and can in no way be considered an endorsement from the trademark holder.

Tables of Contents

CHAPTER 1. INTRODUCTION 6

CHAPTER 2. WHAT IS A PLANT-BASED DIET? 9

    EAT FULLY ON PLANT FOODS 12
    PLANT FOODS TO BE WHOLE 14
    CARBOHYDRATES SHOULD BE AT THE BASE 16
    DON'T DRINK YOUR CALORIES 18
    MOVE 20
    REASONS TO FOLLOW A PLANT-BASED DIET 23

CHAPTER 3. BENEFITS OF PLANT BASED DIET 27

    REASON NUMBER ONE: LOWER YOUR CHOLESTEROL 29
    REASON NUMBER TWO: HEALTHY ANTIOXIDANTS 31
    REASON NUMBER THREE: HIGH FIBER INTAKE 32
    REASON NUMBER FOUR: ASTHMA BENEFITS 33
    REASON NUMBER FIVE: REDUCE RISK OF BREAST CANCER 34
    REASON NUMBER SIX: REDUCE THE DEVELOPMENT OF KIDNEY STONES 35
    REASON NUMBER SEVEN: REVERSE AND PREVENT HIGH BLOOD PRESSURE AND HEART DISEASE 36
    REASON NUMBER EIGHT: CONTROL AND PREVENT CANCER 37
    REASON NUMBER NINE: DECREASE INSULIN RESISTANCE 38
    REASON NUMBER TEN: REVERSE AND PREVENT DIABETES 38
    REASON NUMBER ELEVEN: OBESITY CONTROL AND WEIGHT LOSS 40
    REASON NUMBER TWELVE: HEALTHIER BONES 41
    REASON NUMBER THIRTEEN: DO IT FOR THE ANIMALS 43
    REASON NUMBER FOURTEEN: DO IT FOR THE ENVIRONMENT 44
    REASON NUMBER FIFTEEN: IMPROVE YOUR MOOD 45
    REASON NUMBER SIXTEEN: SKIN AND DIGESTION IMPROVEMENTS 46
    REASON NUMBER SEVENTEEN: IMPROVE OVERALL FITNESS 47
    REASON NUMBER EIGHTEEN: IT'S SO EASY 48
    POSSIBLE VEGAN SIDE EFFECTS 50

CHAPTER 4. THE PLANT-BASED 21-DAY MEAL PLAN 62

CHAPTER 5. WHY YOU NEED TO TAKE CHARGE OF YOUR HEALTH WITH NUTRITION 67

CHAPTER 6. PLANT -BASED DIET FOR WEIGHT LOSS 73

    DON'T FORGET TO EXERCISE 76
    WELL ORGANIZED MEAL PLAN 78
    UNDERSTAND YOUR BODY 79

GET ENOUGH SLEEP AND RELAX EFFICIENTLY 80
GET PROFESSIONAL SUPPORT 81
CREATE TIME 82
RECIPES 83

CHAPTER 7.   TIPS AND TRICKS 84

CHAPTER 8.   LET'S GO SHOPPING 93

CONCLUSION 108

Chapter 1. *Introduction*

Selecting the perfect diet plan can be confusing thanks to the variety of diet plans available these days. Irrespective of what diet plan you opt for, almost all nutritionists and dietitians across the globe recommend diet plans that limit processed foods and that are based more on whole and fresh foods. The Plant-Based Diet is based on these universally preferred foods.

This introduction is going to clear away all ambiguities and doubts regarding the whole-food, plant-based diet plan and provide logical explanations to the benefits it offers.

The whole-food plant-based diet plan is more flexible and understanding than other diets, too. It is mostly comprised of plant-based foods, but you can also have some animal-based products.

Now knowing that eating animal products is a huge risk to your health, it definitely stands as a solid reason why you should opt for plant-based foods. Besides improving your overall health, these foods have numerous benefits to your body. First, they are rich in fiber. Therefore, your digestion will be improved. Their high fiber content, however, demands that dieters should slowly change their usual meals because the bodies take time to adapt. This is a worrying statistic, especially bearing in mind that obesity is linked to cardiovascular diseases and diabetes. Adopting a plant-based diet can help in promoting weight loss. The great thing about this is that you will lose weight naturally without having to worry about gaining again in the future. Usually, the fad diets that people rush to rely on have long-term negative effects. Most people complain about gaining more weight after they had initially shed some pounds. Eating plant foods could prevent such effects.

A plant-based diet emphasizes the consumption of anything derived from plants - vegetables, cereals, nuts and seeds - minimizing or excluding animal products. While some may think that a plant-based diet is just another term for a vegetarian or even a vegan diet, there is a fundamental difference. Plant-based diets emphasize the consumption of whole and natural foods and avoid processed foods such as tofu, seitan or packaged products, even if they are technically vegan or vegetarian.

A diet composed only of plants will be beneficial in maintaining healthy skin. Providing your skin with the nutrients it requires is the best way of keeping it smooth and glowing. Unfortunately, people lack information about this. As such, they are forced to try different skin products with the hopes of giving their skin a natural glow and clear complexion.

Eating right is a solution to almost every disease that we might be suffering from. We have been blinded by the media from realizing that the cure we need is in our food choices.

Chapter 2. *What is a Plant-based diet?*

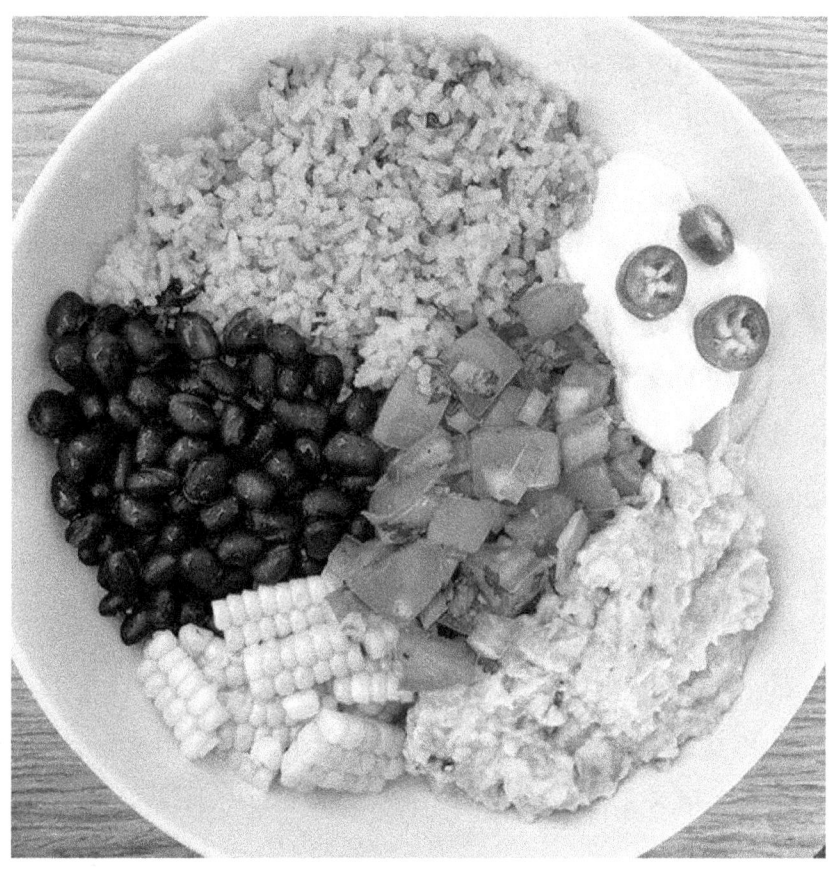

Plant diet is a term that comes from the English plant-based diet, which would have to be translated as a plant-based diet. It evokes obvious associations with veganism, but do these terms really mean the same thing?

Veganism is often understood as a whole lifestyle that includes the fight to reduce animal suffering, pro-animal activism, and attitudes associated with it. A plant-based diet is, in this respect, a much narrower concept, limited only to diet. There are a few minor differences. A plant-based diet does not have to be 100% plant-based. May allow small amounts of meat, fish, or dairy products. However, veganism does not allow this possibility. On the other hand, the plant-based diet should be health-oriented and based on low-processed products, while veganism is not necessarily the case. Many vegans like to eat unhealthy products if they were prepared without the participation of animal components.

To sum up - the plant diet assumes that most calories come from plant products that are low-processed and composed in the diet so as to promote good health and may or may not be a vegan diet.

Plant-Based Vs. Vegan & Vegetarian
In some major ways, vegetable-based diets are different from vegan or vegetarian diets. Vegans and vegetarians

that eat foods that are refined packaged, and may not even end up eating a healthy diet.

Someone who follows a plant-based diet can choose to eat vegan or vegetarian and may or may not use animal products. Some people who follow a generally plant-based diet can consume some products of animal origin, but they include a very small portion of their diet.

Eat fully on plant foods

Eating real food that grows from earth is the most important thing. Most likely, the reason people don't eat enough plant-based food is that they still don't realize how strong plant nutrients are in maintaining our health. Most people still feed on the flesh and products of other animals, not because there is something so natural, necessary or rational about it, but primarily because the major marketing share in supermarkets, stores, and food advertising are occupied by meat, animal, fast, processed and packaged products. Vegetable foods without salt, sugar, and refined fat still account for only a small percentage of the food industry's profits.

At the same time, it is the complete plant foods that are proven to have the most healing effect on our bodies. Cardiovascular disease, diabetes, obesity, osteoporosis, asthma, gout, and any chronic illness have an indisputable link to nutrition, lifestyle, and physical activity. And that's good news. All we need to do is be empowered enough to choose the right foods and live actively.

Vegetable food is at the heart of any healthy diet. Plants are the natural repositories of chemical elements assembled under one sheath in their most complete and complete form. They contain all the vitamins, minerals, antioxidants, isoflavones, essential fatty amino acids, and all other yet-to-be-tested phytonutrients that can sustain the life and health of all of us. Every breakthrough in medicine, any medicine that is used to suppress the symptoms of an illness as a result of an unhealthy lifestyle, contains active ingredients derived from a plant or chemical element synthesized on the basis of one already existing in a plant. Therefore, eating plants is the first and most important condition for living in health and well-being. Everyone has a very intimate, emotional, and even addictive relationship with the food they eat. Therefore, the task of vegans is not only to teach compassion for animals and the care for nature that is irreversibly destroyed by industrial animal husbandry but also to break the dependence of most people on aggressively advertised animal and processed products. People's true connection to food is that of plant food.

Plant foods to be whole

Eating only plant food is not enough to stay healthy. Everyone is a complete organism made up of whole cells. That is why all of our cells need the most comprehensive food we can provide. Whole plant foods mainly include fruits, vegetables, grains, and legumes in their least processed and natural state. Nuts and seeds are also part of an entirely plant-based diet, as are mushrooms (though not plants), spices, and all green leaves. Eating whole foods restricts or excludes processed and extracted substances such as extracted fats, sugars, and proteins. This means as much as possible without extracted oils, no added sugar, and artificial sweeteners, no superfood packets of powders, or protein shakes. Eating whole foods does not mean catching and eating an entire onion without cutting it, nor eating as a raw eater. The idea here is not to deprive the ground food of its essential components, such as fiber, phytonutrients, antioxidants, etc. Removing fiber from fruits and vegetables, for example, raises blood sugar levels, and the consumption of extracted fats causes the blood plasma to become greasy, and the arteries clog. Of course, this also means eliminating packaged foods whose content label is a whole lesson in chemistry. Whole-grain flours, edible milk or fermented foods as tempeh are not technically whole foods since in the process of processing some of their substances are lost, but from a health point of view, they are much closer to whole foods than bottle fat, protein isolates or sweeteners such as glucose-fructose syrup. Many foods can be vegan, but at the same time, they are excessively concentrated sources of salt, sugar, and fat. So, when we talk about eating whole foods, we do not mean absolutely excluding everything that is not food in its entirety but to adjust in the most convenient way for us to base from vegetable sources of carbohydrates, fats, and proteins in there at least a processed form.

Carbohydrates should be at the base

In addition to the need for whole foods, our cells need, above all, sufficient energy. The main source of energy in the human body is food, which, when eaten, is broken down into its main nutrients - carbohydrates, fats, proteins, and water. Of these, it is the carbohydrates that make the cells draw on their glycogen supply, the fuel that makes our body's engine run at full speed.

All whole plant foods contain a full supply of these macronutrients. There are no plants that contain any of them. However, the difference is in their percentage in each food. Fats and proteins are also extremely important for our physical and mental health. However, in order to have a balanced diet, carbohydrates must be the highest percentage of the substances we take with our food. The basis of good nutrition in healthy people with normal physical activity is that about 80% of the total calories a day comes from carbohydrates, 10% fat, and 10% protein. This is the best ratio of foods with which the body can completely metabolize glucose. This diet is the most natural thing for a man. The world's healthiest nations, including the Bulgarian people, have historically eaten the largest number of carbohydrate-based plant foods. Potatoes, corn, different varieties of wheat, millet, rice, buckwheat, all kinds of fruits and vegetables. Popular low-carb diets for weight loss may indeed have a quick effect, but with prolonged exercise, they pose serious health risks. The problem with blocked blood vessels does not exist only with meat and animal products. Even coconut oil, oil, and olive oil can cause blood to become greasy and blockage of the artery walls with a plaque of fat. Fat accumulation prevents glucose metabolism, so if you eat carbohydrates from whole grains, fruits, and vegetables, but continue to gain weight, then the problem is not the carbohydrates, but the fat accumulated in your blood vessels from before. So, if someone is going for carbohydrate plant foods, I recommend first doing at least one week of healing cleansing to clear the fat and plaque accumulated before starting eating the right foods in the required amounts. Before we get to the right food, it is a good idea to create the necessary prerequisites for its absorption and for our body to get used to the new regime.

Don't drink your calories

Drinking them is one of the easiest ways to burn excess calories in your body. We now know that a statistically significant number of people may be drinking between 800 and 1200 calories a day from morning coffee or distemper, from coca-cola, energy drinks, or cappuccino to work, from the beer with friends afterward, or a glass of wine before going to bed. The problem is, our brains don't even register those calories as calories. Like any other creature on the planet, one does not need to drink anything but water to be healthy. If you still want to drink coffee, drink it clean - no added sugar. If you make herbal tea, drink it without any additional sweetener. In just a few days, you will notice how much more saturated and fresh you will feel. It is known that digestion begins in the mouth when we are salivating. The more food is chewed, the better it is metabolized. I'm also a fan of juices, especially carrots, but it's a good idea not to discard the garbage fibers, but at least put some in the cup of juice. If you stop eating your calories, you will immediately feel how much more energy you will have throughout the day. Most of these drinks contain large amounts of sugar and other sweeteners that instantly raise blood sugar, followed by an equally dramatic drop. This insulin reaction becomes even more dangerous when we add to the fact that we drink these fast carbohydrates without fiber and ballast in minutes and even seconds. This means that we will have a quick burst of energy within minutes of drinking the sweetened beverage, but that will come back to us like a boomerang, and we will head down in the early afternoon. On the other hand, when we eat slow carbohydrates from whole foods, they contain a large amount of fiber, which regulates the smooth distribution of blood sugar and the flow of energy to our cells, so that we are constantly alert and fit.

Move

Proper nutrition is not the whole story when it comes to human health. Just as we need a balance between nutrients for the body to function most optimally, so do we need a balance between diet, movement, and other lifestyle-related factors.

In addition to the storage of nutrients in whole plant foods and herbs, exercise also plays a preventative role in protecting us from cardiovascular disease, hypertension, diabetes, obesity, osteoporosis, protecting us from colds, infections, and depression. Physical activity improves functions of blood circulation, lungs, skin and muscle tone, healing of wounds, and lowering of bad cholesterol.

If you improve your diet, physical activity becomes a must. Without physical exertion, most people on a particular diet regain their weight loss or revert to their old lifestyle. Restricting calories or eating only once a day causes the body to store calories in the form of fat instead of burning them. The body prepares for an emergency of calorie deficiency, so it saves most of it as a supply. Therefore, a lifestyle that involves an abundance of whole foods high in slow carbohydrate foods that is physical activity-oriented and movement is much more likely to bring fat burning, good figure, and health in the long run.

In the first 10 minutes of moderate physical activity, the body burns carbohydrates, which are stored as glycogen in the muscles. With continuous movement and physical activity, the body begins to rely less and less on glucose and burns fatter. Trained muscles develop a much better ability to burn fat than untrained, and the more muscle you have in proportion to your body fat percentage, the more efficiently the food is metabolized to its nutrients.

The time to recover and rest after physical activity is the period when muscles are built. The type of exercise determines the size and shape of the muscles. For example, if you ride a bicycle, you will have more developed muscles in your legs and thighs, while, for example, one tennis player may have a much more developed leading arm than the other. However, as you can guess, the type of food also plays a very important role in building the physique.

A slow carbohydrate diet is most effective as carbohydrates from whole plant foods are the main and best source of glycogen for our cells. Physical activity dramatically increases the flow of oxygen, so foods rich in antioxidant vitamins A, C, and E are extremely important in the process.

In general, vitamins and minerals play a key role in releasing energy and restoring the body. Red beets and all green leaves are very valuable helpers in building red blood cells that transport oxygen to the muscles. Raw fruits, vegetables, seeds, and nuts are extremely important for building connective tissue and joints that are stressed in all kinds of physical exercises.

Reasons To Follow A Plant-Based Diet

1. Improve Your Health Status

Over the past 5 years, scientific articles that show the benefits of increasing the consumption of plant-based foods have not ceased to be published, articles that indicate that following a more plant-based diet helps prevent and even reverse some of the diseases that they cause more incidences of deaths in the western world, being in many situations more effective than medication or surgical interventions.

This type of plant-based diet is the only one that has been shown to reverse the number 1 cause of deaths - heart attacks. Doctors such as Dean Ornish and Caldwell Esselstyn proved with their studies that they follow a low-saturated vegetable diet, rich in complex carbohydrates and basically vegetable-based protein, and changing some lifestyle habits (moving the body at least 30 min/day) cardiovascular diseases can be reversed.

A vegetable-based diet also helps prevent certain types of cancer, reduces the incidence of heart disease and diabetes, cholesterolemia, hypertension, Alzheimer's, Parkinson's disease, rheumatoid arthritis, ulcers, and vaginal infections.

A plant-centered diet has a positive effect on the prevention of accumulation of abdominal fat, the appearance of acne, aging, allergies, asthma, body odor, cellulite, eczema, metabolic syndrome, and body weight control.

With just increasing the consumption of fruits and vegetables, we increase the chances of extending our life expectancy, but a life with a higher quality of health. On the contrary, the consumption of meat and other foods of animal origin, such as dairy products, have shown that possibly due to its high content of saturated fats, arachidonic acid, and Heme iron, life is shortened.

The consumption of meat, fish, dairy, and eggs also increases exposure to antibiotics, mercury, and other heavy metals and xenoestrogens in fish and carcinogenic substances in meat that are formed when cooked at high temperatures.

Contrary to popular belief, most vegans get enough protein in their diet, consume more nutrients than the average of omnivores, and usually maintain an adequate weight. There are only two vitamins that we cannot find in plant foods, these are vitamin D, which we get from sun exposure, and vitamin B12, produced by micro bacteria that live on earth, and from which one should be supplemented.

2. Maintain Your Proper Weight

The evil of many is the accumulation of weight that one adds up over the years, from the age of 22, the only thing that can grow is a belly or a tumor. So, to prevent the birth of both follows, a vegetable diet will be our ally.

The reality is that if we consume many vegetables in our dishes, the caloric intake of these will decrease since, on average, a cup of vegetables gives us between 10-50 kcal. And if above, we are replacing with these ingredients other fatty, sweet, and processed foods, you will undoubtedly be reducing the calories consumed at the end of the day, and you will even feel fuller since you will consume more fiber.

3. Eat Healthy And Economical

Many people believe that eating healthy or plant-based foods is expensive, and they turn to processed food or junk, "fast food" because they believe it is the most economical. Certainly, this is not reality.

Visiting a fast-food restaurant such as Burger King and/or Mc Donald's to buy hamburgers, fries, and sodas will not be cheaper than buying 1 package of lentils, 1 package of rice, 1 onion and a bag of frozen spinach with what you can prepare a delicious and complete stew for the whole family.

The only thing you save by consuming these junk food restaurants is time, cooking time. But believe me that once you get into the kitchen, you can prepare twice as many servings, freeze them, and you have them for other days of the week. It's just about being practical and sometimes a little creative, playing with different spices, seasonal vegetables, and different cereal or legumes.

Lentils, beans, and peas are some of the most economical and high nutritional value foods you can find in the supermarket. When we talk about fruits and vegetables, we should always go for the options that are in season, and even buy extra when they are on sale and freeze them for when it is not their time. So, I do with blueberries and other fruits of the forest, to have a proper reserve of local production in winter.

Chapter 3. *Benefits of Plant Based Diet*

While starting a plant-based diet is an excellent idea and has many wonderful benefits let's be honest, you are mostly here to benefit yourself. I am not here to judge! It is fantastic that you are deciding to put you and your health first! You deserve to be the best version of yourself, with a little bit of legwork, you will be there in no time!

To some people, a plant-based diet is just another fad diet. There are so many diets on the market right now, why is plant-based any different? Whether you are looking to lose weight, reverse disease, or just love animals; the plant-based diet can help you out in a number of different ways! On this diet, you will become healthy on the inside and healthy on the outside.

A plant-based diet is so much more than just eating fruits and vegetables. This is a lifestyle where you are encouraged to journey to a better version of yourself. As you improve your eating habits, you will need something to do with all of your new-found energy! It is time to gain control over your eating habits and figure out how food truly does affect our daily lives! Below, you will find the amazing benefits a plant-based diet has to offer you.

Reason Number One: Lower Your Cholesterol

Let me start by asking you a question; how much do you think one egg affects your cholesterol? One egg a day could increase your dietary cholesterol from 97 to 418 mg in a single day! There was a study done on seventeen lacto-vegetarian college students. During this study, the students were asked to consume 400kcal in test foods along with one large egg for three weeks. During this time, their dietary cholesterol raised to these numbers. To put it in perspective, 200 to 239 mg/dL is considered borderline high.

The next question you should be asking yourself is what is considered a healthy amount of cholesterol? The answer is zero percent! There is no tolerable intake of trans fats, saturated fats, nor cholesterol.

All of these (found in animal products) raise LDL cholesterol. Luckily, a plant-based diet can bring your cholesterol levels down drastically. By doing this, you will be lowering your risk of disease that is typically related to high cholesterol levels.

The good news here is that your body makes the cholesterol you need! There is no need to "get it" from other sources.

Reason Number Two: Healthy Antioxidants

As of recently, there has been a push with products showing they are incredibly healthy due to the fact they contain antioxidants.

These are fantastic as antioxidants help prevent the circulation of oxidized fats that are building up in your bloodstream. As you consume more antioxidants naturally in your plant-based diet, this can help reduce inflammation, lower your blood pressure, prevent blood clots, and decrease any artery stiffness you may have.

To put it into perspective, a plant can contain about sixty-four times more antioxidants compared to animal products such as meat. In the chapter to follow, you will be learning more about the foods that contain antioxidants and how to incorporate them into your diet. The good news is that these foods are healthy, natural, and delicious all at the same time!

Reason Number Three: High Fiber Intake

As you begin a plant-based diet, you will be getting more fiber in your diet naturally. You may be surprised to learn that on average, about ninety percent of Americans do not receive the proper amount of fiber!

This is bad news for a majority of people as fiber has some very good benefits. Fiber has been shown to reduce the risk of stroke, obesity, heart disease, diabetes, breast cancer, and the risk of colon cancer!

On top of these benefits, fiber also helps control blood sugar levels and cholesterol levels.

Reason Number Four: Asthma Benefits

According to the Centers for Disease Control and Prevention, about ten percent of children in 2009 has asthma. This means that in 2009, more children than adults had the risk of having an asthma attack. Asthma is defined as an inflammatory disease.

The question is, what is causing the rise of asthma? You guessed it; it's all in the diet! According to one study, both eggs and sweetened beverages have been linked to asthma.

On the other hand, fruits and vegetables both appear to have a positive effect on lowering asthma in children that eat at least two servings of vegetables a day. In fact, their risk of suffering from an allergic asthma attack was lowered by fifty percent!

Reason Number Five: Reduce Risk of Breast Cancer

While it can be hard to pinpoint the development of breast cancer, it seems there are three steps to creating a healthier lifestyle to lower your risk of developing it in the first place. First, you will want to maintain a normal body weight. Luckily, this can be achieved by consuming a plant-based diet.

On top of eating your fruits and vegetables, you will also want to limit your alcohol consumption. By doing this, individuals have been able to reduce their risk of developing breast cancer by sixty percent!

To put this into perspective, meat eaters have a seventy-four percent higher risk of developing breast cancer compared to those who eat more vegetables. I'm not sure about you, but that just doesn't seem worth it to me!

Reason Number Six: Reduce the Development of Kidney Stones

Did you know that by eating one extra can of tuna a day can increase your risk of forming a calcium stone in your urinary tract by a whopping two-hundred and fifty percent? The risk is calculated by studying the relative probability of forming a stone when high animal protein is ingested.

The theory behind this is that urine needs to be more alkaline if you want to lower your risk of developing stones. When meat is consumed, this produced acid in the body.

On the other hand, beans and vegetables both reduce the acid in the body, leading to a lower risk of developing kidney stones; science!

Reason Number Seven: Reverse and Prevent High Blood Pressure and Heart Disease

Unfortunately, one in three Americans has high blood pressure. Studies have shown that as a diet becomes plant-based, this grants the ability to drop the rate of hypertension. In fact, there is about a seventy-five percent drop between an omnivore and a vegan!

It appears as though a vegetarian diet sets a kind of protection against cardiometabolic risk factors, cardiovascular disease, as well as overall total mortality. When compared against a lacto-ovo-vegetarian diet, plant-based diets seem to also have protection against cardiovascular mortality, type-2 diabetes, hypertension, as well as obesity!

This is fantastic news, especially when you lean that just three portions of whole-grain foods seem to significantly reduce the risk of cardiovascular disease in middle-aged people.

This is the same benefit that a symptom-reducing drug can give you!

Reason Number Eight: Control and Prevent Cancer

To start this little section off, I will inform you that fat from animals is often associated with the risk of developing pancreatic cancer. In fact, for every fifty grams of chicken consumed on a daily basis, your risk of developing pancreatic cancer increases by seventy-two percent!

At this point in time, pancreatic cancer is the fourth most common death-causing cancer in the world. It's pretty simple to avoid if you simply switch your beef to beans!

On the other end of the spectrum, it appears that by consuming 70g of more beans a day can cut your risk of developing colon cancer by seventy-five percent. This may be due to IP (6) which is found in cereal and beans. It appears this plays a major role in controlling tumor-growth, metastasis and preventing cancer. In addition to these benefits, IP (6) overall seems to enhance the immune system, lower elevated serum cholesterol, prevent calcification and kidney stones, as well as reducing pathological platelet activity within the body. That seems pretty nifty for eating just a few more beans and less meat!

Reason Number Nine: Decrease Insulin Resistance

Our bodies are very delicate machines. When fat begins to accumulate in your muscle cells, this interferes with insulin. When this build up happens, the insulin in the body is unable to bring the sugar out of the blood system that your body needs for energy. Unfortunately, high sugar intake makes this situation even worse and can clog your arteries altogether. When you eliminate meat from the diet, this means you will have less fat in your muscles. By decreasing these levels, you will be able to avoid insulin resistance in the first place!

Reason Number Ten: Reverse and Prevent Diabetes

I am going to start off with the bad news. As of right now, diabetes is the cause of 750,000 deaths each year. Since 1990, the number of individuals in the United States diagnosed with diabetes has tripled to more than twenty million people. Within this range, you have one-hundred and thirty-two thousand children below the age of eighteen years old who suffer from diabetes. In 2014, fifty-two thousand people were diagnosed with end-age renal disease due to diabetes. Overall, the United States spent a total of two hundred and forty-five billion dollars in direct cost of diagnosing individuals with diabetes. If these numbers seem overwhelming to you, I have good news; plant-based diet can help with this issue. As you learn how to incorporate more vegetables into your diet, the risk of developing hypertension and diabetes drops by about seventy-eight percent.

Reason Number Eleven: Obesity Control and Weight Loss

In a study completed on various diet groups, it was shown that beans typically have a lower mass index compared to other individuals. These people were also proven to be less prone to obesity when they were compared to both vegetarians and non-vegetarians. This may be due to the fact that plant-based individuals have lower animal intake and higher fiber intake. When you reduce your caloric intake to lose weight at an unhealthy level, this has the ability to lead to unhealthy coping mechanisms such as bulimia and anorexia. As you learn how to follow a plant-based diet, you will be filling up on healthy foods such as vegetables, fruits, nuts, and whole grains. At no point on this diet should you be starving or wishing you could eat more. All of the food you will be consuming are typically low in fat and will help with weight loss.

Reason Number Twelve: Healthier Bones

One of the common misconceptions around a plant-based diet is that due to the fact you will no longer be drinking cow's milk, you will be lacking the calcium your bones need to grow strong. While we will be going over this further in depth later, all you need to know now is that it simply is not true. While on a plant-based diet, you will be receiving plenty of essential nutrients such as vitamin K, magnesium, and potassium; all of which improve bone health. A plant-based diet helps maintain an acid-base ratio which is very important for bone health. While on an acidic diet, this aids in the loss of calcium during urination. As you learned earlier, the more meat you consume, the more acidic your body becomes. Luckily, fruits and vegetables are high in magnesium and potassium which provides alkalinity in your diet. This means that through diet, you will be able to reduce the bone resorption. Along the same lines, green leafy vegetables are filled with vitamin K that you need for your bones. Studies have shown that with an adequate amount of vitamin K in your diet, this can help reduce the risk of hip fractures. Along with these studies, research has also shown that soy products that have isoflavones also have a positive effect on bone health in women that are postmenopausal. By having a proper amount of isoflavones, this helps improve bone mineral density, reduce bone resorption, and helps improve overall bone formation. Overall, less calcium loss leads to reducing your risk of osteoporosis, even when calcium intake is low!

Reason Number Thirteen: Do it for the Animals

Whether or not you are switching to a plant-based diet for reasons other than health, it never hurts to be kind and compassionate toward other sentient beings. At the end of the day, sparing someone's life is going to be the right thing to do, especially when they never asked to be brought into this world in the first place. Unfortunately, this is the whole reason behind the dairy and meat industry. In all honesty, there is nothing humane about taking lives or animal farming. Of course, this goes beyond meat products. There are also major issues with the egg and dairy industry where dairy cows are forcefully impregnated and then have their calves taken away so we can steal their milk. These animals have feelings and emotions just like we do, what gives us the right to use them for their worth and then throw them away like garbage when we no longer have a use for them? Do the animals a favor and eat more plants, it will be better on your conscious. Along with these same lines, you never know what is going to come with your animal products. There are a host of toxins, dioxins, hormones, antibiotics, and bacteria that can cause some serious health issues. In fact, there is a very high percentage of animal flesh that is contaminated with dangerous bacteria such as E. coli, listeria, and Campylobacter. These are all tough to find some time because these bacteria live in the flesh, feces, and intestinal tracts of the animals. With the bacteria being tough to find and kill, this eventually can cause food poisoning. Each year, the USDA has reported that animal flesh causes about seventy percent of food poisoning per year. This means that there are about seventy-five million cases of food poisoning a year, five-thousands of which result in death.

Reason Number Fourteen: Do it for the Environment

We were given this one planet to live on, and we should be doing everything in our power to help protect it. During these trying times, it seems that half of the population believes in climate change while the other half thinks of it as fake news. As a plant-eater, it is our duty to do our part in saving the environment. Unfortunately, the meat and farming industry is going to be a hard beast to take down. Depending on the source, it has been proven that the meat industry is behind anywhere from eighteen to fifty-one percent of man-made pollution. This puts the farm industry ahead of transportation when it comes down to the contribution of pollution to the greenhouse effect. In one pound of hamburger meat that you are consuming, this equals about seventy-five kg of CO_2 emission. Do you know what produces that much CO_2 emission? Three weeks from using your car! Do your part, eat more plants and save the planet.

Reason Number Fifteen: Improve your Mood

When you are making an impact on saving the animals and saving the environment, it is no surprise that your mood will enhance! As you begin to cut back on animal products, you will be abstaining from the stress hormones those animals are producing while they are on their way to the slaughterhouse. This factor alone will have a major impact on your mood stability. By eating plants, this helps individuals lower their levels of fatigue, hostility, anger, depression, anxiety, and overall tension. The mood boost may be due to the antioxidants mentioned earlier in this chapter.

On top of these added benefits, it seems as though carbohydrate-rich foods like rye bread, steel cut oats, and brown rice all seem to have a positive effect on the serotonin levels in the brain. Serotonin is very important in controlling mood which is why a plant-based diet may help treat the symptoms that are often associated with depression and anxiety.

Reason Number Sixteen: Skin and Digestion Improvements

You may be surprised to learn that skin and digestion are actually connected! If you suffer from acne-prone skin, dairy may be the culprit behind the issue! If you have bad acne, try a plant-based diet. As you eat more fruits and vegetables, you will be eliminating fatty foods such as oils and animal products that may be causing the acne in the first place. On top of this, fruits and vegetables are often rich in water and can provide you with high levels of minerals and vitamins. By consuming more fiber in your diet, this helps eliminate toxins in your body and boost digestion. When this happens, it could clear up your acne!

Reason Number Seventeen: Improve Overall Fitness

Amazing things will happen as you lose weight and clean yourself from the inside out. When people first begin a plant-based diet, there is a common misconception that a lack of animal products means a lack of muscle mass and energy. Luckily, the opposite is true. It seems as though meat and dairy are both harder to digest. When these products are harder to digest, this means that it is taking more energy to do so. As you consume more fruits and vegetables on a plant-based diet, you will be amazed at how much added energy and strength you will develop.

On top of these benefits, a plant-based diet provides you with plenty of great quality proteins if you are looking to build muscle mass. While eating legumes, nuts, seeds, green vegetables, and whole grains, you will easily be consuming the forty to fifty grams of protein per day that is recommended. Of course, this number will vary but depending on your goals; you will easily be able to consume plenty of protein on a plant-based diet.

Reason Number Eighteen: It's So Easy

When you first begin a plant-based diet, you should just expect your friends and family to doubt your life choices. You will be amazed to learn just how easy it is to live plant-based in the modern age. At the grocery store alone, there are incredible plant-based options for you and your family. There are plenty of plant-based milk options, ice creams, mock meats and more. In fact, the alternative sales in the market are expected to each about five billion dollars by 2020! Along with supermarkets, more restaurants are choosing to provide plant-based options as well. Now, you are no longer forced to cook at home if you wish to live this lifestyle. With each passing day, becoming a plant-based person is become much easier compared to earlier times.

Along with it becoming easier, it is also an economical choice. As you narrow your food choices down to seasonal fruits, vegetables, seeds, nuts, beans, and grains, you may be surprised to learn how much you will be cutting down your monthly food expenses! One of the best parts of whole foods is that you can buy them in bulk! When you purchase your foods this way, you will be spending less in a day and less on eating out. Luckily, there are plenty of options for eating plant-based on a diet. We will be going more in depth later in the book, be sure to stick around!

Possible Vegan Side Effects

Much like with any choices we make in our lives; there are always going to be benefits and downfalls. I don't want you to jump into a plant-based lifestyle thinking that everything is going to be perfect and dandy. While yes, there are some amazing benefits that come along with fueling your body properly, there is always the risk of possible side effects. Below, we will go over some of the side effects you should be watching out for.

Side Effect Number One: Energy Issues
As you begin your new diet and begin eating more plant-based, without even realizing it, you will be consuming fewer calories! This is due to the fact that most plants have a lower calorie density compared to the foods that are derived from animals. For most people, this means that you will have to eat more food in order for you to receive the calories your body needs to function. For some, this is awesome! For others, this can be a very difficult task at hand.

Unfortunately, undereating will put you at risk of some health issues. In order to avoid this issue, you may want to track your food intake for a couple of days when you first get started. You may feel like you are eating a lot of food, but often times the calories just won't add up the same. Luckily, these foods will be providing the proper antioxidants, minerals, and vitamins you need to energize yourself so you will not be lacking in that department!

Along the same lines, individuals have claimed that when they switch to a plant-based diet, they feel very sluggish. If you begin to feel this way, it could mean that you are either undereating or you are not eating the proper foods to fuel yourself efficiently. Remember that there is a lot of plant-based junk food. While yes, these are within the diet restrictions, this does not mean that they are any better for you than fries and a burger from your favorite fast food joint.

So, what is the game plan if you feel you are losing energy when you switch to a plant-based diet? You will need to take a good, hard look at the foods you are putting into your body. I want you to make sure that the foods you are choosing are whole. These foods will need to be eaten at a higher volume in order to obtain the nutrition and energy you need. As you do this, be sure to avoid all oils and processed sugars. If you complete this, you should have much more energy and feel better than before!

Side Effect Number Two: Cravings

Changing your dietary habits is not going to be an easy task. Unfortunately, we are typically habitual creatures; this meaning that our bodies like the routine of what we do and what we like. Our taste buds are the same exact way! As you change your diet to more vegetables and fruits, you should expect to have cravings for non-plant-based foods. This is especially true if you are not eating enough (see side effect number one) or your body simply wants a certain calorically dense food.

One of the best ways to overcome cravings is to not get wild and crazy with your diet change if you are just getting started. Instead of cutting everything cold turkey, take reasonable steps to remove your favorite foods from your diet. As you do this, you will want to find foods to replace these favorites with. Luckily, there are plenty of healthy and delicious alternatives to help get you past your cravings. Do you want something sweet? Try coconut ice cream or even rice milk chocolate! As you begin to distance yourself from unhealthy, processed foods, I promise you will begin to crave them less!

To help overcome cravings, I suggest you set yourself up for success! The first step will be to remove all temptation from your home. This way, when you reach for your old habits, they won't be at your disposal. Once this is complete, find plant-based versions of your favorite foods. Eventually, your taste buds will adjust to your new way of life, and you may be surprised what healthy foods you will begin to crave!

Side Effect Number Three: Digestive Issues

More than likely, you saw this coming the moment you read that a big part of this diet is beans; we all know the poem about beans! As you begin a plant-based diet, you may begin to experience an uncomfortable feeling in your stomach after your meals. I want to go ahead and say now that you cannot blame the food! Our bodies adjust to food depending on what we eat, and the bacteria found in our gut will optimize itself to digest whatever it needs whether we are eating processed junk or healthy whole foods.

As you begin to change the composition of food from animal products to vegetables, legumes, and grains, you may be changing slightly too sudden for your body. Unfortunately, this has the potential to lead to bloating, diarrhea, or even constipation. Why you ask? Fiber.

Fiber is an indigestible part of plants that for the most part, are not typically found in processed foods nor animal products. However; fiber is crucial for the body's ability to digest food properly and our overall health. In fact, fiber is the reason we are able to move the junk of our food out, so we become, ahem, regular.

Along with becoming more regular, fiber also will help you lower your risk for chronic disease and aids the body in nutrient absorption. Yes, you will be using the bathroom more, but this is actually a really good thing. Eventually, your body will transition to the new food and will get over the digestive distress. As your digestion becomes smoother, you will no longer have stomach pains, and you will actually begin to feel lighter!

Side Effect Number Four: Social Struggles

As mentioned earlier, many people will doubt your new diet choice. We happen to live in a very carnist society where many of our meals revolve around meat. Think about this for a second; what do you typically eat at a baseball game? Hamburgers and Hot Dogs? You go out to your favorite restaurant; what do you typically order? More than likely, this meal revolves around meat with the vegetable on the side! As you switch over the more plants, set yourself up for success by expecting a backlash.

When people first start off with a plant-based diet, this can be a true test for individuals. You may be shocked to learn how many of your friends are suddenly "nutritionist" and will tell you about everything you are missing out on by not consuming animal flesh. While it may be hard to hear, I suggest you never allow anyone to keep you from living your life the way you want.

While it may be difficult to go out with friends now, that does not mean that it is impossible. As mentioned earlier, the world is becoming more plant-friendly as we continue to evolve and change the meaning of what it is to be plant-based. At the end of the day, it does not matter what anyone says to you or what they think of your life choices. You are very well aware of the incredible benefits this diet has to offer you, and that is all that matters! Instead of fighting back when the small comments come, simply prepare yourself and be ready to answer all stupid and legit questions that revolve around a plant-based diet. Those who truly care for you will understand.

Potential Nutritional Shortfalls

When you begin a plant-based diet, you will need to be mindful about your essential nutrients. On a plant-based diet, there are a few potential nutritional shortfalls if you are not careful about what you are eating on a daily basis. Some of these missing vitamins and minerals will be essential if you wish to continue a proper body function. Below, we will go over some of the more popular shortfalls plant-based individuals run into. The hope is that by being mindful from the beginning, you can avoid the issue in the first place.

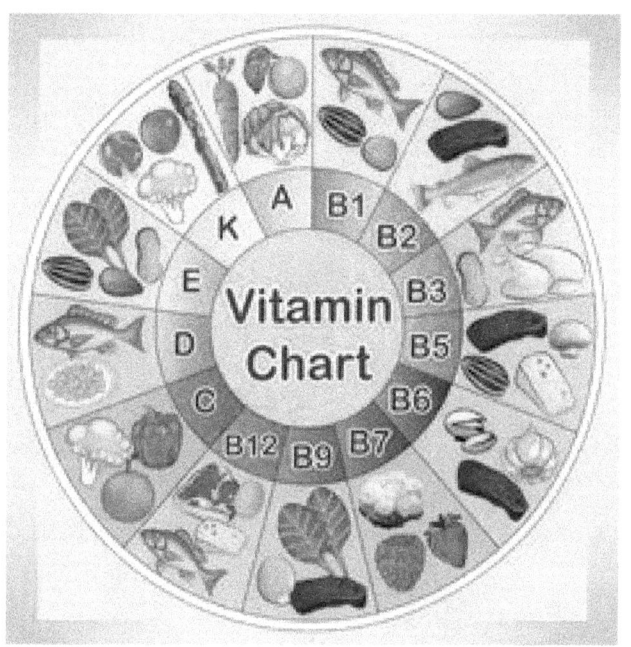

Vitamin B12

If you become deficient in vitamin B12, you enter the risk of bone breakage, elevated levels of homocysteine, abnormal neurological symptoms and anemia. B12 can be found in a number of different foods such as nutritional yeast, seaweed, B12 fortified foods, and soy drinks. As we age, the absorption of vitamin B12 begins to deteriorate. Due to this fact, it is normally advised to take a vitamin B12 supplement.

Vitamin D

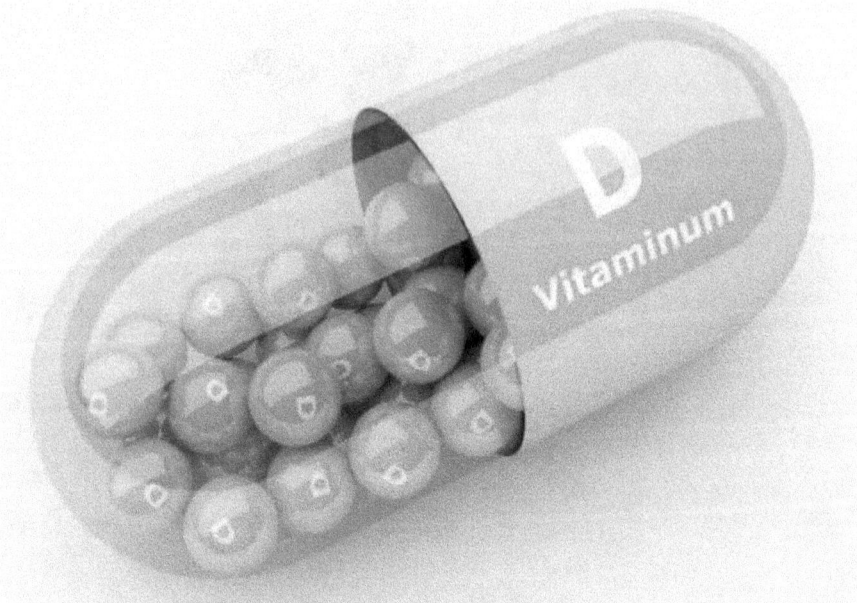

In general, a plant-based diet has been known to low in vitamin D. When you are low in vitamin D; this could mess with the absorption of calcium in your body. As a result, this could potentially lead to brittle bones. It is suggested you expose yourself to a proper amount of sunlight or consider taking a supplement to help meet your requirements. On top of this, you can also consume foods such as juice, rice milk and soy beverages that have been fortified with vitamin D.

Calcium

As mentioned earlier, calcium is going to be a

shortcoming while on a plant-based diet, especially if you typically get your calcium from cow's milk. Instead, you will want to begin consuming dark green leafy vegetables to get your calcium in. Other food sources would include calcium-fortified breakfast cereals, soy beverages, and even calcium. This will help grow strong bones and keep you healthy overall.

Iron

Iron is another supplement that will be vital on your plant-based diet. This is very important for the formation of red blood cells within your body. In order to avoid deficiency of iron, you can consume iron-fortified foods like dry fruits and dark green vegetables. It should be noted that plant-based iron is typically less absorbable by the body compared to those on a meat-based diet. While not impossible, it is harder.

Protein

Protein is a big factor that we will be going over later in this book. There are many individuals who feel it is impossible to get a proper amount of protein on a plant-based diet, but it simply is not true. There is no need to consume eggs, dairy products, and meat to get the proper amount of protein. You can find protein in nuts, seeds, legumes, whole grains, and other vegetable proteins.

Zinc

Finally, we have zinc. Zinc is important in the diet as it helps build a healthy immune system. As you switch over to a plant-based diet, it should be noted that you will have higher concentrations of phytates in your body, making the absorption of dietary minerals slower compared to a meat-based diet. This can be helped by eating zinc-rich foods like legumes, nuts, whole grains, and even pumpkin seeds.

There are a number of different reasons you should make the dive and switch to a plant-based diet. While there are downfalls, you can see that there is always a solution. I am not saying that a plant-based diet is meant for everyone, but it certainly doesn't hurt to try! After all, you are just eating healthier, and it doesn't hurt that you are helping animals and the environment along the way. I hope that at this point, you are convinced to make the switch to becoming a healthier version of you. Once you have a grasp on these foods, I will also be providing you with some of my favorite plant-based recipes along with a grocery list to make it even easier! Be prepared to be mind-blown on just how delicious eating plant-based can truly be.

Chapter 4. *The Plant-Based 21-Day Meal Plan*

Week 1 Meal Plan

Day 1

Breakfast: Creamy Chocolate Shake

Lunch: Sniffle Soup

Dinner: Rustic Pasta

Day 2

Breakfast: Hidden Kale Smoothie

Lunch: French Lentil Soup with Paprika

Dinner: Vegan Lasagna

Day 3

Breakfast: Blueberry Protein Shake

Lunch: Squash Soup

Dinner: Garlic Alfredo Pasta

Day 4

Breakfast: Raspberry Lime Smoothie

Lunch: Chickpea Lentil Soup

Dinner: Golden Pasta

Day 5

Breakfast: Peppermint Monster Smoothie

Lunch: Beans and Lentils Soup

Dinner: Creamy Spinach Pasta

Day 6

Breakfast: Almond Banana Granola

Lunch: Quinoa Salad

Dinner: Haka Noodles

Day 7

Breakfast: Eggless Omelet

Lunch: Devilish Ramen

Dinner: Veggie Stir Fry

Week 2 Meal Plan

Day 1

Breakfast: Polenta

Lunch: Basil Noodle Salad

Dinner: French Potato Salad

Day 2

Breakfast: Lemon Apple Breakfast

Lunch: Kale Salad

Dinner: Grilled Mushrooms

Day 3

Breakfast: Oats and Chia Bowl

Lunch: Penne Pasta Salad

Dinner: Sweet Potato Noodles

Day 4

Breakfast: Grilled Tofu

Lunch: Tofu Noodle Bowl

Dinner: Brown Rice Stir Fry

Day 5

Breakfast: Grilled Pineapple

Lunch: Teriyaki Stir Fry

Dinner: Sweet Potato Hash

Day 6

Breakfast: Hot Grilled Watermelon

Lunch: Garlic Alfredo Pasta

Dinner: Roasted Chickpeas

Day 7

Breakfast: Creamy Chocolate Shake

Lunch: Baked Sesame Fries

Dinner: Niçoise Salad

Week 3 Meal Plan

Day 1

Breakfast: Winter Refresher

Lunch: Tempeh Bacon Hash

Dinner: Baked Sesame Fries

Day 2

Breakfast: Veggie Breakfast Hash

Lunch: French Lentil Soup with Paprika

Dinner: Vegan Lasagna

Day 3

Breakfast: Pumpkin Smoothie

Lunch: French Potato Salad

Dinner: Garlic Alfredo Pasta

Day 4

Breakfast: Chocolate Avocado Mousse

Lunch: Quinoa Salad

Dinner: Haka Noodles

Day 5

Breakfast: Berry Lime Smoothie

Lunch: Quinoa Salad

Dinner: Teriyaki Stir Fry

Day 6

Breakfast: Banana Green Smoothie

Lunch: Basil Noodle Salad

Dinner Grilled Mushrooms

Day 7

Breakfast: Tempeh Bacon Hash

Lunch: Chickpea Lentil Soup

Dinner: Creamy Spinach Pasta

Chapter 5. *Why You Need To Take Charge Of Your Health With Nutrition*

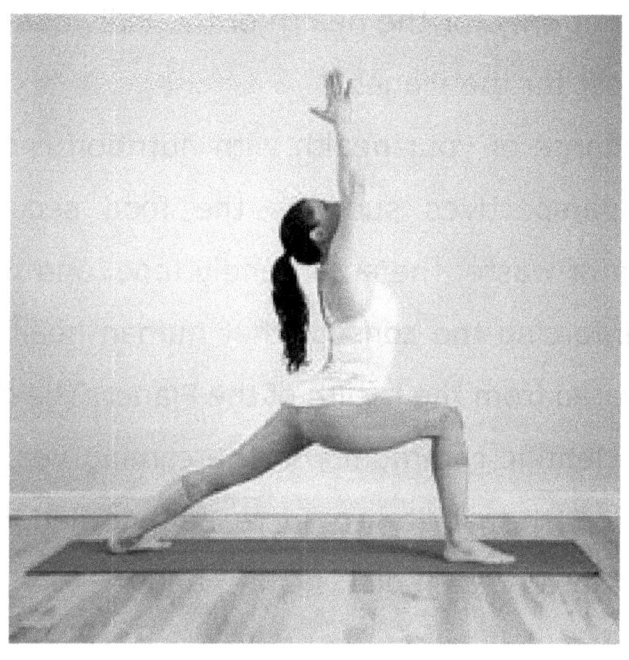

Proper nutrition is a central factor for the well-being of society, especially the western one, characterized by a growing increase in obesity and other related degenerative pathologies. Whenever we consume a high-energy or nutritionally unbalanced meal, we cause postprandial stress in our body, inducing endogenous protection mechanisms that involve the immune system. This condition, if continued over time, can cause obesity and overweight conditions associated with an increase in several metabolic risk factors such as triglycerides, inflammation, insulin resistance, and many others. The excess consumption of these stressful foods represents damage not only for the health of the individual but also a huge cost for the Planet.

Taking charge of your health with nutrition is based on several perspectives such as the food security, the reduction of waste, the eco-friendly food, and functional food, reinforcing the concept that human health cannot be separated from the health of the Planet. The challenge for the scientific community in the coming years will be focused on the ability to increase knowledge of the relationships between diet, health, and the environment.

Your Health with Nutritional Needs

There is no longer any doubt that a balanced diet is the basis of a healthy life. An incorrect diet understood above all as inadequate consumption of food and supply of energy and nutrients, is, in fact, one of the main risk factors for the onset of numerous chronic diseases. Proper nutrition, therefore, passes through an adequate supply of energy, macro and micronutrients, and other elements first of all water.

However, it is now clear that our body's response to food

consumption is susceptible to variability between individuals. In recent years, therefore, the world of scientific research is moving more and more towards a more personalized nutritional approach aimed at bringing maximum benefit to everyone based on individual characteristics. Many studies have shown that our body's response to food consumption varies radically within the population. The factors that define this variability are related to the lifestyle, health status, and genetic characteristics of the consumer.

Very recently, even the so-called intestinal microbiota, that is the population of microorganisms that cohabits in our intestine, and which represents a crucial component in maintaining our health, has been recognized as a fundamental factor in modulating dietary responses. This varies from individual to individual and can transform the components of the diet with which it comes into contact. Different microbiota corresponds to different products of these transformations of nutrients and non-nutrients that we introduce with the diet, with clear individual effects on the state of health.

Healthy nutrition then identifies a dietary approach that is tailor-made to the individual and the entire population, and that develops a set of directions, recommendations, specific products, and services.

Functional Foods and Health

In recent years, numerous studies have shown that diet and lifestyle, together with the environment, are the main causes of longevity. The case of functional foods is defined as any food, part of food, drink or food groups, with additional positive effects on health maintenance, physiological homeostasis, or on disease prevention. Thanks to the progress of food science and technology, in fact, in recent years, traditional foods have appeared on the market, along with traditional foods, capable of providing health-promoting components, generally non-nutritious such as polyphenols, probiotics, prebiotics, that are able to positively and selectively regulate one or more physiological functions of our body.

These foods can be naturally functional, such as fruit, vegetables, and natural cereals, e.g., the tomato for lycopene, olive oil for tocopherols, green tea, and many others or traditional foods, e.g., dairy products, baked goods, and pastries, salad dressings, non-alcoholic drinks. Thanks to their properties, these compounds can contribute to the well-being of the body with various biological activities, such as antioxidant, anti-inflammatory, antihypertensive, hypocholesterolemia, antimicrobial, antiviral, and so on.

It is essential to emphasize that functional foods are neither drugs nor supplements and that their consumption, even if capable of making a concrete contribution to health, must not ignore a healthy lifestyle accompanied by constant physical activity. Bearing in mind its value diet, the quantity, and frequency of consumption, the possible interaction with other foods and drugs, the impact on the metabolism and the risks of allergy.

The Fruits

Fruits contain few calories. Their consumption does not present any health inconvenience, unlike other types of foods. According to some studies, eating several fruits in one day can detoxify the human body.

Fruit consumption also helps to lower cholesterol levels in the body, which helps prevent cardiovascular disease. Even better, high consumption of fruit lowers the risk of infarction or hemorrhage by acting directly on the tension it causes to fall. Like other benefits, it is important to note that fruits contain certain vitamins that act positively on mental health. You will benefit from excellent physical and mental health by consuming a lot of fruit.

The Vegetables

Vegetables are particularly rich foods. They are full of fiber and water. They are also very rich in vitamins and minerals necessary for the proper functioning of the body. Doctors often recommend eating vegetables because they are very rich in antioxidants and contain very few calories, which is excellent for the human body.

The Proteins

Proteins play a vital role in the human body. They constitute a privileged source of energy and strength. They contribute greatly to strengthening muscles, bones, hair, and nails. It is therefore recommended to consume foods that contain such as meat, fish, eggs, cheese, or milk. Be careful about the excesses for these foods!

Chapter 6. *Plant-Based Diet for Weight Loss*

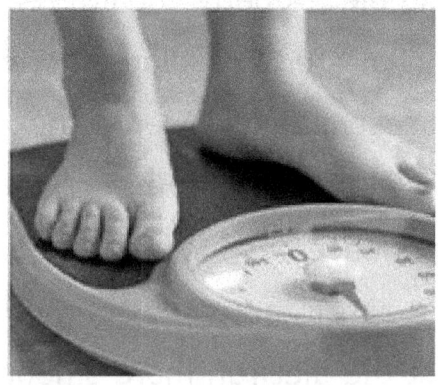

It is a natural fact that only through watching what we eat, will we have the most impact on our weight. This is where the plant-based diet really shines and lets you enjoy automatic, effortless fat burning without all the usual calorie constraints of other diets.

Weight loss is an almost certain result you will enjoy once you start the plant-based diet, but this is not the only benefit that you will enjoy. Think of all those activities you have always wanted to pursue but shelved because you simply had no energy left after your usual day's work.

Well, time to dust off those hobbies and the things you enjoy doing, because on the plant-based, you will have more energy for your daily work and play! The accompanying mental clarity and sharpness of thought are also positive effects which you will have as a direct result of the diet. A better health report card, by way of optimized cholesterol readings, normalized blood sugar and a corresponding lowered risk of cardiovascular diseases are also just some of the beneficial health effects experienced by most on the diet.

This book's aim is primarily to give you the tools with which to let the diet run more smoothly and seamlessly in your daily life. Something that many learn is that a diet is almost only as good as the number of recipes it has in its repertoire. The benefits of a particular diet may be numerous, but if you are forced to have the same stuff every breakfast, lunch and dinner, even the most avid supporter of the lot would probably have problems sustaining the diet. This is where I am most happy to say that the plant-based diet has quite some leeway for the concoction of various different recipes, and it is the purpose of this book to bring you some of the more delicious and easy-to-prepare meals for your gastronomic pleasure!

For the beginners as well as the adepts, the recipes contained within are created specifically to be appealing to your palate while not requiring you to literally spend the whole day in the kitchen! Concise and to the point, the recipes break down meal preparation requirements in a simple step by step format, easy for anyone to understand. An additional 21-day meal plan is also structured to serve both as guidance as well as inspiration for the new and old adherents to the diet.

Don't forget to exercise

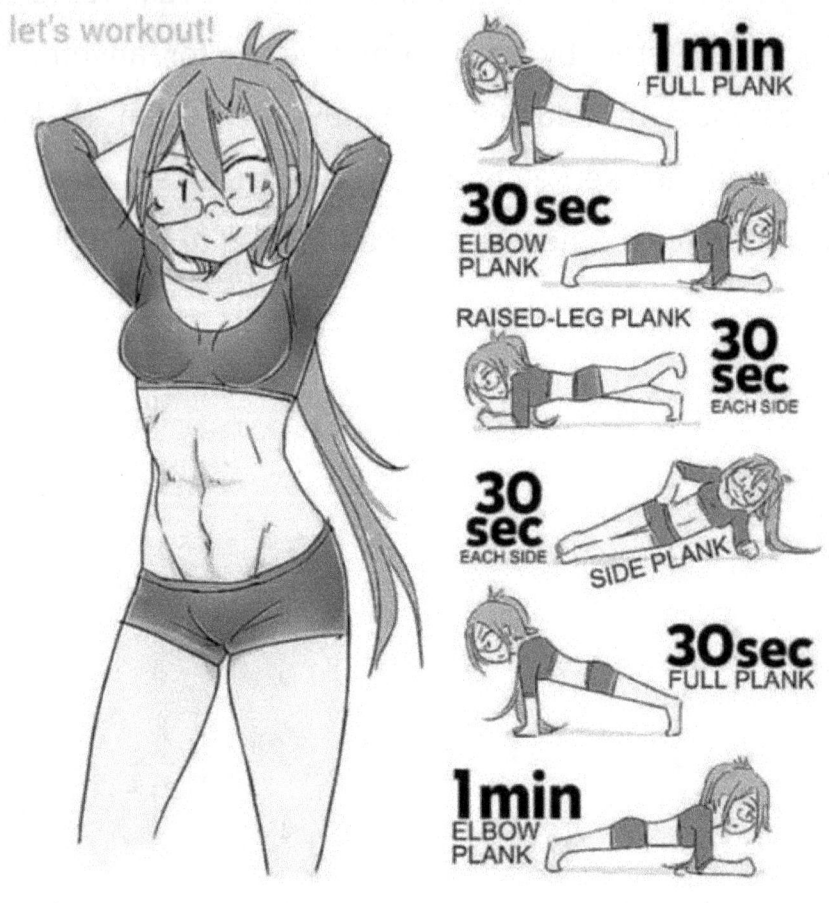

It has always been said that dieting is an effective way to lose weight. However, to keep the weight off, exercise is required. Many studies have shown that exercising while dieting is actually the best way to lose weight. Firstly, the diet becomes more effective and you lose weight faster if you exercise. But it also gets you in the habit of continuing your exercise when your diet is complete.

The exercise expected is not something that is not achievable either. Even with just forty-five minutes of exercise each day, can increase your weight loss by over ten percent! Anything that can get your heartbeat pulsing higher and faster than normal is considered exercise.

Often times, dieting will make you lose weight in many parts that you don't want to lose weight in, such as curvaceous or softening lines. Studies have shown that combined with exercise, dieting can help reduce your body mass index, waist circumference, and percentage of body fat.

Another concern is that with dieting, often times you appear lighter because your muscle and bone density is reduced. That is not a healthy lifestyle in the long term. Exercising will stimulate the growth of your muscles and have your body burn the fat instead of your metabolic tissues.

It is also important to understand that the idea behind dieting is that most people want to look skinnier and overall better. However, lean is what will make you look perfect! Being lean will highlight your figure and keep your body healthy and toned. Skinny means that you have lost a lot of muscle density and water retention. In the long run, it can affect your calcium, iron, and zinc levels in your body.

Kick-starting your weight-loss journey

To get things done the right way and to ensure your body benefits from this diet, it is essential to consider the following things prior to starting this regimen

Well Organized Meal plan

Please note that the main purpose of this book and diet plan is to help you lose weight and help in maintaining a healthy lifestyle. Because of this, you have to follow a strict plan to achieve your goals. This book provides a 21-day plant-based plan to kick-start your wellness journey. Please remember that this meal plan will require some commitment, and it is not how your diet will always be structured after the 21-day plan. After 21 days, once your body has adjusted, you will be able to make a consistent meal plan schedule where fasting is not required.

Understand Your Body

Getting your blood tested for the existence of any underlying condition is important to ensure that you start the regimen without worrying about it affecting your health negatively. Though, it doesn't harm your body, but in case you are suffering from a serious condition, it is best that you don't go on any sort of weight loss diet. It is important to get your blood tested for lipid panel, liver and kidney function, inflammatory markers, thyroid panel and blood count.

Get enough sleep and relax efficiently

It is important that you understand that you must take this diet easy and relax while practicing it. Your goal must not be to quickly cut down your carb intake, so you can lose an enormous amount of your body weight as soon as possible. Rather, you should reduce it slowly and gradually. Don't worry; you will still benefit a lot from this plan. Going easy on yourself helps you experience less side effects and enables your body to adjust comfortably to the completely new diet plan.

Get Professional Support

It is wise to get the assistance of a professional healthcare practitioner, dietician, or nutritionist who can help you out in preparing good meal plans for you. In this case, this e-book will do this job for you by providing you with more meal plans and guidance in the next series. Nonetheless, it is a good idea to consult a professional at least once before commencing the diet just to make sure that you know your body is ready for it. You will also find it easier to prepare good meal plans that are customized just for you.

In case, you suffer from heart diseases or other conditions such as epilepsy, HBP, diabetes (TYPE 2), Alzheimer's or any other medical condition, then it is absolutely essential for you to get a professional's help before and during the plan.

Create time

This is one of the most crucial factors to consider before implementing the low-carb diet. You must not start it when you are going through an extremely hectic schedule and have no time to spare for yourself. This is because this diet demands you to prepare special meals and get used to different foods that you aren't accustomed to eating regularly. These changes will stress you out, so you need to have enough time to devote to this new routine, at least for about two weeks.

Therefore, you must start the plant-based diet when you are emotionally, psychologically, and physically relaxed and free.

Be careful with other people's opinions

If you are to achieve optimal this goal, you will definitely need to understand that you cannot just eat anything even when in social places otherwise you will end up jeopardizing your entire regime since it takes time for any carbs you take to be completely out of your body. As such, you should be psychologically prepared to take different foods that might attract some attention and well-meaning but often misleading comments about the diet. Being prepared will ensure you don't give up.

Recipes

By now, you should have enough info to start your plant-based diet plan. In the subsequent chapters, we will discuss what your eating schedule should look like throughout your first four weeks of starting. This will ensure you start the diet correctly and be well on your way to losing excess weight quickly and eating healthy. This book comes with more than 50 pre-designed ketogenic diet recipes to get you started! There's a recipes section after the weekly diet plans, so keep reading.

Chapter 7. *Tips and Tricks*

Before we send you on your way to your new healthy lifestyle, there are a few important tips and tricks for you to learn and keep up your sleeve. In the beginning, it always seems easy to begin a new diet. You have this new found motivation and energy to change your life. But, what happens when that energy burns out in a few weeks? By knowing some tips and tricks about the plant-based diet, these will keep you going when times get rough!

Getting Started on a Plant-based Diet

1.   Find Your Motivation

Truly, I cannot express the importance of this enough! If you are here in this book, there was probably something drastic that made you want to make a major change. This reason is your why and what you should set your goals around. Whether you are looking for mental clarity, more energy, or helping a disease, always try to remember why you are starting this lifestyle in the first place. For bonus points, write down your why on a sheet of paper so that you can look at it when you need added motivation.

2. Remember to Eat

As mentioned earlier, a plant-based diet is very filling when you are consuming whole foods. It will be important that you remember to eat more than you are used to. Luckily on a plant-based diet, you can say goodbye to counting calories. Now, you can fill up on salad, fruit, quinoa, beans, and even baked potatoes to your heart's content! The whole point of this diet is to live off the good food, and over time, the body adjusts to the volume of food. After a while, you will learn to rely on your satiety cues and natural hunger.

3. Prepare Food

As you start a plant-based diet, I encourage you to take a stroll through your kitchen. In the beginning, you will begin to recognize the foods that may not be as beneficial to you as a whole food. I suggest you toss these foods or give them away, so you keep yourself out of temptations reach. Instead, fill your fridge and pantry with healthy foods such as beans, rice, and potatoes! This way when you get cravings for unhealthy foods, there won't be any in your house!

4. Take it Gentle

Switching over to a plant-based diet does not need to happen overnight! Instead, I suggest taking a gentler approach and slowly switch your diet to become more plant-based. If you make sudden changes, you could potentially feel restricted and ultimately cheat yourself out of your amazing diet. An example would be to use avocado instead of butter! While it is a change, it will take some time to get used to. As you increase the healthy plant-based ingredients in your life, you will slowly eliminate the bad stuff.

5. One Meal at a Time

There are no rules saying that being plant-based needs to be a now or never type of deal. Instead, try switching one meal at a time to be more plant-based. One of the easier meals, I have found, is breakfast! Instead of your normal milk and cereal, give oatmeal with your favorite fruit a try! There is also delicious avocado toast or breakfast potatoes! I highly suggest trying some of the recipes provided in this book to help you get started! Slowly, you can switch all of your meals to being plant-based, and soon it won't even be a second thought.

6. Find Good People

I mentioned earlier that many people close to you will doubt your lifestyle choice, but there are also many likeminded people out there in the world that are going through the same changes as you. Typically, it is easier to go through changes when you have company to share your struggles and successes with. It is a fantastic idea to form a support group so you can reach out for help and inspire others. I suggest checking out internet forums or even Facebook groups for you to connect with. Just remember that you are never alone on this journey!

7. Keep it Fun

Switching to a plant-based diet is not meant to be a form of torture. I hope that eventually, you learn to enjoy your food choices and perhaps even look forward to it. Luckily with modern technology, you have recipes at your fingertips. There are always new foods to try and recipes to give a shot. A good way to keep your diet fun is to have an adventurous side. The next time you visit the grocery store, I challenge you to choose out a fruit or vegetable that you have never heard of before. When you have made your selection, use the internet to find ideas on how to cook this item. You may be surprised at what you learn about food and about yourself!

8. Commit

As you begin the plant-based diet, the best thing you can do is make the commitment to yourself. There are a number of reasons people begin the plant-based diet. Why are you here? Why do you feel a plant-based diet can change your life? At the end of the day, it does not matter what anyone else thinks. If you want to make this commitment to yourself, you make this commitment! It is time to take your health into your own hands. You are the only one who can make health decisions for yourself, make sure those decisions are the best ones possible. You owe yourself that much.

Plant-based on a Budget

One major excuse individuals use not to eat healthily is that they feel eating healthy can be too expensive. The trick here is to make smart choices. There are plenty of ways to strip the diet down to the basics; whole foods can actually be easily affordable for just about anyone! All you need is some knowledge about whole foods, and you will be able to fit all of your nutrients into your budget with ease!

1. Stay Home!

This seems like a given but eating at home instead of going out to a restaurant can save you a lot of money whether you follow a plant-based diet or not! Instead of dining out several times a week, eat out for an occasional treat! If you are constantly on the move and rely on fast food, begin to prepare snacks in advance. This way, you will have full control over your meals and what goes into them. Also, by staying home, this will give you a fantastic chance to work on those cooking skills!

2. **Choose Whole Foods**

While this may seem like a given, whole foods are going to be some of the cheapest staples you can buy! Luckily, the whole foods are going to offer the most essential nutrients as well! Some of the more popular, budget-friendly foods include brown rice, oats, potatoes, carrots, leafy greens, frozen vegetables, apples, oranges, other fruits in season, and all of the beans and lentils!

3. **Think Big**

Not literally, but when you buy food in bulk, you can get much more bang for your buck! When you are at the grocery store, look for the big packages or family packs. Typically, these will provide better value compared to smaller bags or containers. In this case, you will want to pay special attention to the unit price located on the price tag; this number will tell you the cost per pound. By following this rule, you can choose the cheapest option.

4. **Keep it Simple, Stupid**

If you are just starting the plant-based diet, there is no reason to get crazy and wild in the kitchen! Just because you are switching your diet, this does not mean that you need to become a crazy, skilled chef. Keeping your meals simple does not mean that they are going to be boring. As you can tell from the recipes earlier in this book, recipes can be easy and delicious at the same time. Often times when you use too many ingredients, this makes it tough on the pallet and your digestion tract. Do yourself a favor and start small. As you get better with this lifestyle, that is when you can experiment a bit more with your meals.

5. Buy in Season

This is vital when it comes to shopping for a plant-based diet on a budget. The good news is that food that is grown in season is cheaper and tastes much better. In the winter, keep an eye out for citrus fruits and root vegetables. In the summer, you can keep your eyes out for nectarines and watermelon. Do yourself a favor and visit your local farmers market to get the freshest produce possible. You may be surprised to learn the wide variety of food that is made available to you!

6.   **Frozen**

Lastly, frozen fruits and vegetables. These items are typically cheaper and can be very convenient. Frozen fruits and vegetables are typically picked once they are ripe and then frozen right away; this meaning that the foods will maintain their nutrition. This is a fantastic idea, especially in the winter when fresh produce may be limited on variety and quality. Just remember to read the label of ingredients so you can avoid any added butter, sauce, or seasoning.

Chapter 8. *Let's go shopping*

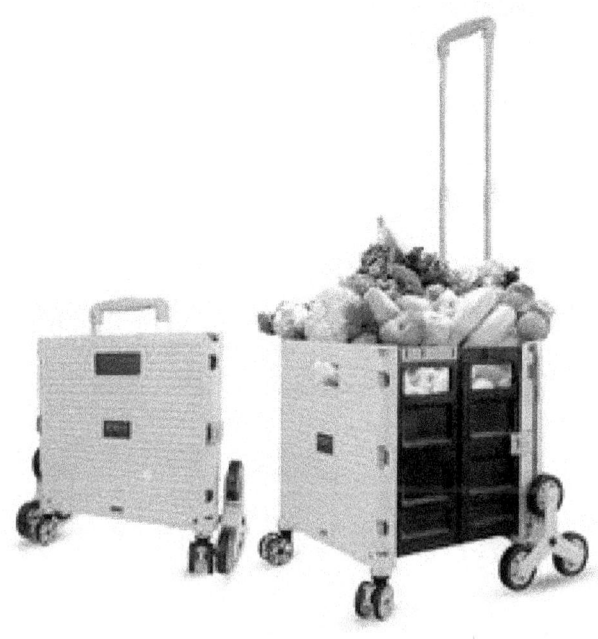

Now that we have a good understanding of the nutritional value of plant-based foods, let us go to the supermarket to stock the cupboards, fridge, and freezer with everything we need to get this new lifestyle started.

Every supermarket is laid out in a similar way, so this list will be designed to make it as easy as possible for you to get what you need and navigate the layout with ease. There will always be a fresh produce section which usually is the first area you come across but is sometimes the last. It is always to one side of the supermarket. The dairy fridges are usually close by to the produce, along with the vegetarian fridges. The health foods aisle will be adjacent to the produce section along with the bulk bins.

The middle aisles of the supermarket are always reserved for convenience and junk foods, cereals, and packet meals. The personal care and cleaning products follow the rice, pasta, canned foods, and baking supplies, then comes the freezer aisles and bakery. Let's begin!

FRESH PRODUCE

Anything in this department is available to you as it is all fruits and vegetables. Take your time getting to know each area from the berries to the citrus, root vegetables to the leafy greens. It is recommended not to overwhelm yourself at first, so stick to what you know and every visit, pick up something you haven't tried before and given it a go. You'll find new favorite foods and ones you don't like so much, but it's all part of the fun!

FRUIT

Citrus fruits: Lemons, oranges, limes, grapefruit, mandarins.

Stone fruits: Peaches, plums, nectarines, cherries, apricots

Melons: Watermelon, honeydew, cantaloupe

Berries: Strawberries, raspberries, blueberries, blackberries, gooseberries, kiwi

Tropical fruits: Banana, mango, pineapple, papaya, dragon fruit, lychee, coconut, passionfruit

Apples and pears: Granny Smith, Braeburn, golden delicious, red delicious, pink lady, gala, Fuji, McIntosh.

Dates and figs: you will find fresh in the produce aisle.

VEGETABLES

Roots: Potato, sweet potato, yam, carrot, beets, celeriac, radish, parsnip, ginger, turmeric, turnip.

Bulbs: Garlic, onion, shallots, green onion.

Stems: Celery, asparagus, rhubarb.

Marrows: Pumpkin, acorn squash, spaghetti squash, gem squash.

Cruciferous: Broccoli, cauliflower, Brussel sprouts, cabbage.

Leafy greens: Lettuce, spinach, collard greens, chard, arugula, kale, bok choy, watercress.

Peppers: Bell, chili, jalapeno, habanero, banana pepper.

Other: Mushrooms, cucumber, zucchini, eggplant, tomato, cherry tomato artichoke, avocado, beans, peas, corn, sprouts.

FRESH HERBS:

Leafy herbs: Basil, cilantro, parsley, mint.

Cooking herbs: Marjoram, oregano, sage, thyme, rosemary, anise, caraway, bay leaves, kaffir lime leaves.

Accompaniment herbs: Dill, chives, fennel, lavender.

DRIED FOODS

These foods are mainly fruits, herbs, and spices and also apply to the bulk bin sections, which are a great way to try new foods and flavors without paying much money or worrying that you'll be stuck with a huge amount of something you won't like.

Nuts: Almonds, brazil nuts, cashews, hazelnuts, macadamias, pecans, pistachios, pine nuts, walnuts.

Seeds: Chia seeds, flax seeds, flaxseed meal, hemp hearts, sesame seeds, sunflower seeds, pumpkin seeds, hemp hearts.

Dried Fruit: Apricots, dates, figs, mulberries, cranberries, raisins, blueberries, banana chips, mango, goji berries, shredded coconut, desiccated coconut.

Dried Herbs: Basil, celery seed, cloves, coriander seeds, dill, Italian herbs, oregano, parsley, rosemary, sage, thyme.

Dried Spices: Black pepper, cardamom, chili powder, chili flakes, cinnamon, cumin, curry powder, garlic powder, nutmeg, onion powder, paprika, turmeric.

Salt: Sea salt, pink Himalayan salt, black salt.

Dried legumes: Black beans, chickpeas, red kidney beans, white kidney beans, pinto beans, lentils, cannellini beans.

Other: Nutritional yeast, kelp flakes, dried seaweed, nori sheets, rice paper rounds.

CANNED FOODS

This aisle is a haven for a vegan with so many whole food options that can be kept in a pantry for emergencies, additions to meals and has a very long shelf life. Obviously fresh foods are better for you but rotating canned foods into your diet will help ensure you have enough options to keep you happy on this new lifestyle.

The following is a recommended list of handy and delicious items that work well in recipes. If you have a favorite canned vegetable or fruit that is not on this list, please continue to enjoy it.

Vegetables: Diced/chopped tomatoes, tomato puree, corn, pumpkin puree, beets.

Fruits: Coconut milk, coconut cream, peaches, pears, pineapple, apples, jackfruit.

Legumes: Black beans, lentils, red kidney beans, white kidney beans, pinto beans, chickpeas, cannellini beans, butter beans, bean salad, vegan refried beans (caution as a lot of refried beans contain pork lard)

JAR GOODS:

Often better than canned goods due to being stored in glass rather than tin. There are many amazing food items in this area that should be kept and savored in your fridge or pantry. They are often richer in flavor than their fresh counterparts and marinated in herbs, spices, and oils that complement meals very well.

Vegetables: Olives, sundried tomatoes, pickles, banana peppers, roasted red peppers, salsa, sauerkraut, capers, artichoke hearts.

Fruit: Applesauce, high-quality whole jams or spreads.

NUT AND SEED BUTTERS

You won't be sorry you found this aisle. These butters are full of concentrated proteins, fibers, and vitamins and are essential to recipes at any meal of the day from smoothies to satays to desserts.

Nut Butters: Almond butter, cashew butter, hazelnut butter, peanut butter, peanut and coconut butter, macadamia butter, walnut butter.

Seed Butters: Pumpkin seed butter, sunflower seed butter, tahini.

GRAINS

Grains can be found in multiple areas of the grocery store. The cheaper items can be found in the bulk section, the higher priced items will be found in the health food aisle and they can also be found in the baking aisle. It is recommended that you take your time finding the brands and types that work for you, but if you are trying something for the first time, start in the bulk section.

Rice: White rice, brown rice, wild rice, basmati rice, jasmine rice, long grain rice, short grain rice, saffron rice.

Pasta: Linguine, spaghetti, penne, macaroni, lasagna, cannelloni, shell pasta. (most of these can be found in whole wheat varieties to up the nutrient factor and there are also very good gluten-free pasta brands now too)

Oats: Rolled oats, quick oats, steel-cut oats.

Grains: Amaranth, bulgur wheat, barley, couscous, quinoa, buckwheat, millet.

Other: Popcorn.

BAKING AND COOKING

There are many items in this aisle that are essential to creating dishes to help you recreate favorite meals from before this transition. There are also a lot of processed and refined items that are damaging to your health. Do your best to choose the whole-grain, raw and whole varieties as much as possible.

Flour: All-purpose, almond, buckwheat, chickpea, coconut, whole wheat, rice flour.

Baking: Arrowroot powder, tapioca starch, potato starch, corn starch, baking powder, baking soda, agar-agar, cocoa powder, cacao powder.

Sugar: Raw sugar, brown sugar, coconut sugar, blackstrap molasses.

Sweeteners: Maple syrup, agave syrup, stevia.

Other: Vegan chocolate chips, vegan cooking chocolate, cacao nibs, vanilla extract.

SAUCES, OILS, AND CONDIMENTS

One of the most important aisles for cooking vegan meals. There are many ethnic and cultural items that you may have never heard of before but are packed with flavor. Be cautious of fish sauce or seafood ingredients in Asian sauces and flavorings.

Vinegars: Balsamic vinegar, red wine vinegar, white wine vinegar, rice wine vinegar, apple cider vinegar, malt vinegar.

Oils: Avocado oil, olive oil, coconut oil, sesame oil, peanut oil, sunflower oil, hemp oil, flax oil, walnut oil, canola oil, coconut cooking spray.

Condiments: Ketchup, Dijon mustard, yellow mustard, whole grain mustard, vegan mayonnaise, sriracha, hot sauce, sweet chili sauce.

Sauces: Soy sauce, coconut amino, tamari (gf).

Others: Miso Paste

FREEZER SECTION

A great place to find staple items that come in very handy when you've run out of fresh produce or want to keep something fresh that you use often.

Vegetables: Mixed, peas, carrots, corn, spinach, broccoli, cauliflower rice, avocado

Fruit: Mixed berries, blueberries, raspberries, strawberries, blackberries, smoothie mix, mango, banana, cranberries, cherries.

Meat Substitutes: Vegan mince, vegan burger patties, vegan chicken filets.

Other: Phyllo pastry, puff pastry (just check the ingredients for oil instead of butter)

CHILLED SECTION

Some supermarkets keep the vegan items next to the dairy items, whereas other supermarkets will keep the vegan fridges next to the fresh produce. Take your time getting acquainted with your own supermarket.

Milk: Almond milk, coconut milk, cashew milk, rice milk, oat milk, hemp milk, soymilk.

Cheese: Vegan sour cream, vegan cream cheese.

There are many great vegan kinds of cheese out there ranging from soy cheese to nut cheese. There is also a great variety of types from shredded, blocks, creams, and slices.

Yogurt: Coconut yogurt, almond yogurt, soy yogurt, cashew yogurt.

Butter: Vegan margarine (used as margarine and also for cooking and baking)

Meat substitutes: Veggie burgers, breakfast patties, vegan sausages, deli slices.

Other: Silky tofu, extra firm tofu, coconut water, orange juice.

BAKERY

Lots of goodies in this section that are not what you want in your cupboard or that contain dairy or eggs. If you stick to the edges of this section and avoid the cases, you should navigate yourself quite easily.

Bread: Sourdough loaf, rye bread, multigrain bread, unsliced bakery loaf, baguettes, bagels, English muffins. (some bread contains egg or milk so check the labels)

Wraps: Large tortilla, mini tortillas, corn tortillas.

OTHER:

Extras that are usually found in the health food aisle.

Vegan protein powder

Vegan protein bars

Spirulina

Greens powder

TIPS AND TRICKS AT THE GROCERY STORE:

The number one hardest thing about going vegan can be a sense of loss. We are creatures of habit and we get used to having the things we like, so when these things are taken away and not replaced with something else, the sense of grief will derail our commitments and see us reaching for what we promised ourselves we would give up.

So, how do we avoid this from happening when going vegan? You've already accomplished the first part which is educating ourselves on why we are giving up the meat, dairy and eggs and positive reasons for how doing so will improve our lives.

The second part is to make sure we don't feel like we've given anything up. The best way to do this is by taking a hard look at your previous diet. Write down what your favorite meals are, what you would take for lunch, what you would have for breakfast every day, and most importantly, what were your favorite treats. Once you have this written down, try to find reasons as to why you have chosen these foods and meals. Is it because they taste good? Or remind you of something? Do they make you feel a certain way when you're done? Full, or satisfied, energized or guilty? Once you've figured this part out, you might begin to understand your relationship with food a little better.

Now, we need to find vegan replacements for these meals and food items that will replicate these feelings, so you never feel like you're missing out.

For example:

You usually have a fried egg and white toast with butter for breakfast because it's quick to make and fills you up and is simple. You might really enjoy switching to avocado toast instead. The avocado will mimic the egg and butter in fat content, and a sprinkle of hemp or chia seeds on top will help to replace the protein from the egg. You could switch your white toast for a good quality whole wheat toast that will keep you fuller for longer but still takes the same amount of time to make. A sprinkle of nutritional yeast will and sea salt with black pepper will keep it tasty and you happy.

You only eat tuna salad sandwiches for lunch with a packet of chips. Switch the tuna salad for a chickpea salad that you can make ahead of time. Make sure you have a delicious soft whole wheat bread or bun to satisfy the carb side of this equation. Find a good quality root vegetable chip to tide you over while you slowly switch this to a nut and seed snack mix and maybe some sliced veggie sticks.

Your afternoon snack is always yogurt and chocolate biscuits. There are fantastic coconut or almond yogurts out there now! Try a few to find a good replacement that has a similar taste to your old favorite. Maybe trade your chocolate biscuit for a trail mix that has some pretzels and vegan chocolate chips in there.

You adore chips and dip and can't imagine giving that up at night while you watch TV. Okay! Maybe keep the chips for now but sub the dip for homemade guacamole or hummus. Slowly incorporate veggie sticks and delicious seed crackers into the mix as you slowly pull the chips out of your nighttime routine.

As you can see, there are so many ways to trick yourself into a new diet and lifestyle. Please just be patient with yourself, love yourself for trying to be healthier, and keep reminding yourself of all the good that is about to come your way with this new way of being.

Conclusion

The plant-based diet in reality isn't a tough one to practice. To me, it comes across as the easiest way to diet for food preparation and digestion. Plant foods cook the fastest and are easy to grasp for beginner cooks.
While there might be arguments as to the plant-based diet being a vegan, vegetarian, plant to animal-based, or a partially processed foods diet, the plant-based diet stands as a unique one by itself. It combines and eliminates aspects of all four of these ways of eating to create a wholesome approach that serves the body better.

In my opinion, it is one that eliminates the presence of animal and processed foods in meals but incorporates plant-foods to the best possible. Now, will you question if these dishes will be tasty? I can guarantee with full backing that the WFPB offers some of the most delicious foods that there are. Think of fresh crunchy salads with super tasty dressings, scrumptious soups that incorporate plant creams, nuts, and seeds for mouthwatering sips, and the list is endless.

While I have found the plant-based diet to be more nutritious than regular diets, it offers tremendous benefits that serves as a proof for longevity too. Counting the benefits, it facilitates weight loss, reduces the risk of heart diseases, cancers, and cognitive decline. In addition, for the high amounts of nutrients present in plant foods, they result in the right nutritional balance within the body.

Beginning the whole foods plant-based diet is as easy as tucking away all the animal and processed foods that you previously enjoyed and replacing them with plant-based options.

It is a fun world with these recipes! I am happy that I can share them with you and look forward to the exciting foods that you make. Don't forget to prep your mind, self, and kitchen in ways that will make it a fun journey for you. Consider the lifestyle as an adventure and take it one step at a time. Also, create a small community of similar dieters that will encourage you on this path. Meanwhile, own your kitchen and make it a paradise for your plant-based food preps. I can guarantee that you will enjoy walking into your kitchen often and you will magically create foods that will leave you wanting more. This Plant-Based Cookbook for Beginners will be your companion for many days to come!

Now, it is time for me to say a goodbye but not quite a goodbye. I am heading out to create my next exciting cookbook on a topic that I know will excite you as much as this. You should look out for it!

www.ingramcontent.com/pod-product-compliance
Lightning Source LLC
Chambersburg PA
CBHW070722030426
42336CB00013B/1893